Post-Baby Passion

Reigniting Sex & Intimacy After Childbirth

Natesa Estella Sparks

ISBN: 978-1-7642608-3-1

This book is intended for educational and informational purposes only. It does not substitute for professional medical advice, diagnosis, or treatment. Always seek the guidance of your physician, midwife, pelvic health therapist, or other qualified healthcare provider with any questions you may have regarding your postpartum recovery, sexual health, or medical condition.

The names and scenarios depicted in this book are purely for illustrative purposes only. Any resemblance to actual persons, living or dead, or actual events is purely coincidental.

The author and publisher disclaim any liability for direct, indirect, or consequential damages arising from the use or application of the information contained in this book.

Table of Contents

Preface

When you have a baby, everyone lines up to give you advice. They'll tell you how to swaddle, how to breastfeed, how to get your newborn to sleep longer than twenty minutes. But here's the part nobody seems to talk about out loud: what happens to *you*. Your body. Your relationships. Your sex life.

It's almost like society gives you a six-week permission slip— "Okay, you're healed now, go back to normal"—and if you don't, you're left wondering if something's wrong with you. The truth? Six weeks is a myth. Healing takes months, sometimes years, and it doesn't just happen in your stitches or your hormones. It happens in your confidence, your identity, and your sense of connection.

This book was born out of listening to countless mothers whisper the same worries behind closed doors. Questions like:

- "Why does sex still hurt months later?"
- "What if my desire never comes back?"
- "Will my partner lose patience with me?"
- "Why do I feel guilty for not being ready?"

If any of that sounds familiar, you're in the right place. This isn't another manual that tells you to just "relax" or "spice things up." (You've probably rolled your eyes at that advice already.) This is a straight-talking, research-backed, and compassion-filled guide to intimacy after childbirth—the kind I wish more women had on their nightstands.

Here's what you can expect as you move through these pages:

- We'll talk honestly about your body after birth—what really happens, not the fairy tales.

1

- We'll get into the emotional shifts that hit you when you're suddenly responsible for keeping another human alive.
- We'll cover pelvic floor rehab, positions that ease pain, and practical ways to rebuild desire.
- We'll go deep into the messy parts too—painful sex, tension with your partner, or the fear that intimacy might never feel the same.
- And because theory alone doesn't change lives, you'll find worksheets, trackers, and reflection prompts at the end of each chapter so you can actually apply what you read.

Now, here's the thing: this book isn't about rushing you. It's not about snapping back or pretending things are fine when they're not. It's about progress, not perfection. Some days you'll move forward, some days you'll backtrack, and all of it is part of the process.

So take a breath. Pour yourself some tea (or reheat the coffee you've already microwaved three times). Settle in. What you'll find in these pages isn't judgment—it's guidance, companionship, and a little humor to keep you going.

Because intimacy after baby isn't just about sex. It's about finding yourself again.

Chapter 1: Knowing Your Postpartum Body

You've made it through pregnancy and childbirth. You may feel proud, exhausted, relieved, or all three at once. But here's the reality: your body has gone through one of the most intense events it will ever experience. And no matter how many Instagram posts tell you that "six weeks and you're back to normal," the truth is far more complicated. Your body is healing, recalibrating, and—let's be honest—sometimes protesting. Let's pull back the curtain on what actually happens, why the timeline isn't as simple as people make it sound, and what you can do to feel more connected to your body again.

The physical reset after birth

First, let's break down the major physical changes:

- **Uterus shrinking**: During pregnancy, your uterus grows from about the size of a pear to the size of a watermelon. After delivery, it starts shrinking back down—a process called involution. Typically, it takes around six weeks, but healing varies. Some women still feel tenderness or abdominal heaviness months later.
- **Hormones crashing and shifting**: Estrogen and progesterone, which were at record highs during pregnancy, plummet almost immediately after birth. This sudden drop can cause mood swings, hot flashes, and vaginal dryness. At the same time, prolactin rises to help you make milk. Prolactin, however, can suppress estrogen—leading to long-term dryness and sometimes low libido while breastfeeding.

- **Pelvic floor recovery**: These muscles, which act like a hammock to hold up your bladder, uterus, and rectum, often get stretched, strained, or torn during pregnancy and delivery. Damage here can mean leaks when you sneeze, pressure or bulging in the vagina, or pain during sex. Without rehab, these issues may persist for months—or even years.
- **Scarring and stitches**: If you had a C-section or vaginal tearing, your body is also healing from stitches and scar tissue. This healing doesn't follow a straight line. Scar tissue can feel tight, sensitive, or even numb.
- **Bleeding and discharge**: Lochia (postpartum bleeding) can last up to six weeks, sometimes longer. While doctors often use this bleeding timeline to decide when sex is "safe," it doesn't account for comfort or readiness.

Now, here's the thing—none of this makes you "broken." It makes you normal. But it does mean that your body has a new baseline, and rushing back into pre-baby expectations only creates frustration.

The myth of six weeks

Here's the traditional script: at your six-week check-up, your OB or midwife says, "You're cleared." Many women hear this as, "You should be having sex now." But clearance simply means your uterus has shrunk, bleeding has stopped, and stitches have healed. It does not mean your body—or your mind—is ready.

Studies show that while 89% of women attempt sex by six months postpartum, up to 83% report pain at first. That means most couples are trying, but most women are also uncomfortable. And here's where the problem starts: when women feel pain but are told they're "fine," they assume the issue is them. It's not. It's the system oversimplifying recovery.

A better model? Think of postpartum recovery like a traffic light:

- **Green light**: You're not bleeding, stitches are healed, and you feel physically comfortable. Sex may feel okay, but don't be surprised if it takes extra lubrication or slower pacing.
- **Yellow light**: You've stopped bleeding but still have discomfort, dryness, or pelvic heaviness. You may need pelvic floor therapy, hormone support, or more time.
- **Red light**: You have ongoing pain, bleeding, or fear about sex. This is a signal to stop and seek help from a doctor or pelvic floor therapist.

The key point: there's no universal "all clear." Six weeks is a milestone, not a finish line.

Expert voices

Here's what professionals say:

- **OB/GYNs** often focus on safety markers: bleeding, stitches, infection, and uterine healing. They tend to give clearance based on these medical boxes being checked.
- **Pelvic floor therapists** look at function: muscle strength, scar tissue mobility, nerve health, and your comfort level. They often see women who were "cleared" at six weeks but still can't have pain-free sex at six months.
- **Sex therapists and counsellors** point out that readiness is emotional as well as physical. Anxiety, body image, and fatigue can shut down desire even if your body has technically healed.

When all three perspectives come together, you get a fuller picture. But too often, women only hear the OB side—and miss the other pieces.

Case example: Maria's story

Maria, 32, had a vaginal birth with a second-degree tear. At six weeks, her OB said she was fine. Maria and her husband tried having sex a week later. She described it as "like sandpaper and fire." She pushed through twice more, then started avoiding intimacy altogether. Her husband felt rejected, she felt broken, and their marriage grew tense.

Finally, Maria saw a pelvic floor therapist. The therapist found scar tissue that needed mobilization and pelvic floor muscles that were clenching too tightly in anticipation of pain. With exercises, manual therapy, and lubricants, Maria gradually regained comfort. Within a few months, intimacy felt good again.

The lesson? Clearance doesn't equal readiness. Support makes the difference.

Gentle self-assessments

You don't need to wait for a doctor to tell you how you're healing. You can check in with your own body safely at home. Here are some ways:

1. **Breath connection**: Lie on your back with knees bent. Place one hand on your belly, one hand on your pelvic floor (between your sit bones). Take a slow breath in. Do you feel your pelvic floor gently expand? Breathe out—

does it relax? If not, your muscles may be holding tension.
2. **Mini Kegel check**: Gently try to squeeze the muscles you'd use to stop urinating. Can you contract and relax fully? Do you feel weakness, shakiness, or pain? This isn't a test of "strength" but awareness.
3. **Scar comfort**: If you have a C-section scar, gently touch the area. Is it tender, numb, or hypersensitive? If vaginal stitches were involved, you can use a clean finger to gently feel around the vaginal opening when you're ready. Any sharp pain or pulling sensation is worth noting.
4. **Lubrication test**: Notice during daily life—do you feel dryness, itching, or discomfort? This could be hormonal, especially if you're breastfeeding, and easily improved with the right support.

These aren't pass/fail tests. They're feedback. And feedback is information you can use to get help early instead of suffering in silence.

Another story: Sara's reality check

Sara, 28, had a C-section. She was shocked to find that her scar felt numb in some places and overly sensitive in others. She hated the way it looked and avoided letting her husband touch her belly. For months she wore loose shirts during sex to hide it. Eventually, in therapy, she admitted that she felt "cut open and damaged."

Her therapist guided her through gentle scar massage, helping her reconnect with sensation. Over time, Sara noticed that the numbness improved and her confidence grew. She realised her scar wasn't a mark of damage but survival. That shift allowed her to let her partner touch her belly again—something small but deeply intimate.

Why this matters for intimacy

Your physical readiness affects not only your comfort but also your confidence. If your body feels weak, painful, or "different," you're less likely to want intimacy. That's not a psychological flaw—it's biology and self-protection. When your body feels safe, your mind opens to intimacy. When your body hurts, your mind shuts the door.

Checkpoint moment

Still with me? Good. Because here's the big takeaway: you're not on anyone else's timeline. Six weeks is just a marker. Pain isn't normal, and you don't have to push through it. Listening to your body now saves you from frustration later.

Key takeaways

- Postpartum healing involves uterus shrinking, hormonal shifts, pelvic floor recovery, and scar healing.
- The six-week clearance is about safety, not readiness for sex.
- Pain, dryness, and fatigue are common and deserve treatment, not shame.
- OB/GYNs, pelvic floor therapists, and counsellors all provide pieces of the puzzle.
- Self-checks help you tune into your healing process.

- Every woman's timeline is unique, and rushing back often causes more harm.

Chapter 2: Emotional Shifts and Identity After Baby

You thought the biggest change would be the sleepless nights, right? And sure, those 3 AM feeds and diaper explosions are exhausting. But ask any new mother what really caught her off guard, and she'll tell you: it was the emotional shift. Because here's the thing—your body heals, but your sense of self? That's a much messier process.

Becoming a mother isn't just adding a new role. It can feel like your old identity was thrown in a blender with your new one, and now you're trying to figure out who comes out the other side. For some women, that transition feels empowering. For others, it feels like loss. And when it comes to intimacy, that loss—of confidence, of freedom, of feeling desirable—can be just as challenging as physical recovery.

So let's talk honestly about how motherhood reshapes your emotional world, why "mom guilt" is so destructive, how fatigue messes with everything, and why mood changes sometimes cross into depression or anxiety.

Motherhood, sexuality, and body image

Pregnancy changes your body in ways you can't always predict. Stretch marks, softer skin, a belly that doesn't snap back, breasts that leak. For some women, these changes feel beautiful—proof of what their body accomplished. For others, they feel like constant reminders that their body is no longer their own.

One study found that over 60% of new mothers reported negative feelings about their body in the first year after birth.

That dissatisfaction is directly linked to lower sexual desire. Why? Because it's hard to feel sexy when you don't feel comfortable in your own skin.

And it's not just appearance. The way your body *feels* can shift, too. If your breasts are sore, or your scar is sensitive, or your pelvic floor feels heavy, your brain sends the message: "Not safe. Not sexy." Your partner may say, "You look beautiful," but if you don't feel it inside, it doesn't land.

Case example: **Nina**
Nina, 35, had twins via C-section. She told me, "I look in the mirror and I don't see me. I see this sagging belly and two scars. My husband says he doesn't care, but I care." For months, Nina avoided letting him see her naked. She'd change in the bathroom, turn off the lights, and keep sex quick and functional. Eventually, she admitted she missed feeling wanted, but couldn't bridge the gap. With therapy, she worked on small steps—standing in front of the mirror without judgement, letting her husband kiss her scar, buying lingerie that made her feel like herself. Slowly, her self-image shifted.

The bottom line? Body image isn't superficial—it's central to how you experience intimacy.

The guilt trap

Now, let's talk about guilt—the invisible weight new mothers carry.

- You feel guilty for not wanting sex.
- You feel guilty for wanting sex when you "should" be focused on the baby.
- You feel guilty for being tired.
- You feel guilty for putting yourself first.

11

This endless cycle is what psychologists call **mom guilt**. It's the idea that no matter what you do, you're falling short. And here's the catch: guilt isn't just an emotion—it's a libido killer. When your brain is running on "I should" and "I shouldn't," desire has no room to show up.

Research shows that mothers who report higher levels of guilt also report lower satisfaction in their relationships. It's not because they love their partners less—it's because guilt crowds out joy.

Case example: **Jasmine**
Jasmine, 29, described it like this: "I'd be nursing the baby and my husband would put his hand on my back. Instead of feeling loved, I'd think, 'I should be giving the baby more attention. I can't give him anything else.' It was like I had no space left for desire."

What helped Jasmine wasn't forcing herself into intimacy. It was reframing guilt. She started reminding herself: "Caring for myself *is* caring for my baby." That shift opened the door to enjoying small moments of touch again.

Fatigue and the body-mind connection

Here's a truth most people underestimate: exhaustion wrecks desire. Not just "I'm a little tired," but the bone-deep fatigue that comes with broken sleep cycles.

Sleep deprivation lowers dopamine and serotonin—neurochemicals that regulate mood and motivation. It also raises cortisol, the stress hormone, which blocks sexual arousal. So when you're exhausted and uninterested in sex, it's not a personality flaw. It's chemistry.

And fatigue isn't just physical. Mental load plays a role, too. Many mothers carry the invisible list: feeding schedules, appointments, baby clothes, housework. By bedtime, your brain is fried. Desire isn't on the menu.

Checkpoint moment: Still with me? Good. Because if you've ever thought, "Why am I so broken?"—you're not broken. You're sleep-deprived. And sleep deprivation changes everything.

Mood changes: normal vs. concerning

Some mood swings after birth are expected. The so-called "baby blues" affect up to 80% of new mothers—tears, irritability, mood dips that come and go. Usually, they resolve within two weeks.

But for about one in seven women, those feelings don't fade— they deepen into postpartum depression. Symptoms include:

- Persistent sadness or hopelessness
- Loss of interest in things you used to enjoy
- Irritability or anger
- Feeling disconnected from your baby or partner
- Anxiety, panic attacks, or obsessive worry

These symptoms directly affect intimacy. If you feel empty, anxious, or numb, sex won't feel appealing. And forcing it only worsens the emotional distance.

Case example: **Laura**
Laura, 27, said, "I love my baby, but I feel nothing for my husband. Not anger, not love—just nothing." She blamed herself for being "cold." In therapy, she was diagnosed with postpartum depression. With treatment—counseling and medication—her

emotional range returned. She later said, "It wasn't that I didn't love him. I just couldn't feel anything until I healed."

The message? Postpartum depression and anxiety are medical conditions, not personal failures. Getting help doesn't make you a bad mother. It makes you a healthier one.

Rebuilding identity

One of the hardest parts of postpartum life is figuring out who you are now. You're still a partner, a friend, maybe a professional, but now you're also "Mom." And society pushes the idea that motherhood should swallow you whole.

But here's the deal: intimacy thrives when you feel whole, not when you erase yourself. Making space for your old self—reading a book, meeting a friend, dressing in clothes you like—isn't selfish. It's essential.

Case example: **Anita**
Anita, 31, told her partner, "I don't feel like myself anymore. I feel like I disappeared." She stopped painting, something she loved, because she thought all her time had to go to the baby. She also avoided sex because she felt like she had no identity outside motherhood. With support, she carved out one hour a week to paint. That small act reminded her she was more than "Mom." Interestingly, her desire for intimacy returned—not because she forced it, but because she started feeling like herself again.

Journaling prompts for self-reflection

Writing can help you untangle the emotional mess. Try these prompts:

- Right now, I see my body as…
- One part of me I miss since becoming a parent is…
- What does intimacy mean to me beyond sex?
- If guilt had a voice, what would it say to me? How could I answer it?
- What small act makes me feel like myself again?

You don't need to share these answers with anyone. Sometimes just writing them out clears the fog.

Practical strategies

- **Name your feelings**: Say out loud, "I feel tired," or "I feel unattractive." Naming emotions reduces their power.
- **Challenge guilt**: Ask, "Would I judge another mom for this?" If not, why judge yourself?
- **Prioritise sleep**: Take shifts with your partner, nap when possible. Sleep fuels intimacy more than effort does.
- **Seek help early**: If sadness or anxiety lingers, don't wait. Treatment works.
- **Protect identity**: Do one thing each week that's just for you. It may feel small, but it's fuel for self-worth.

Checkpoint reflection

So, here's the question: are you giving yourself permission to be both a mother and a woman? Or are you expecting yourself to erase one for the other? Because intimacy lives in that balance— not in perfection, but in allowing space for both.

Key takeaways

- Body image shifts can block desire, but healing your relationship with your body helps intimacy.
- Mom guilt is destructive—it kills joy and desire, but reframing it opens space for pleasure.
- Fatigue and mental load are chemical barriers to desire, not personal flaws.
- Postpartum depression and anxiety affect about one in seven women and directly impact intimacy—but treatment is available and effective.
- Rebuilding identity beyond motherhood is essential for sexual and emotional closeness.
- Journaling and small self-care acts can reconnect you with yourself and your partner.

Chapter 3: Communication After Baby

So here's the scene: you're exhausted, your partner's confused, and neither of you wants to say the wrong thing. He (or she) wonders why intimacy hasn't returned. You wonder why they can't see you're barely hanging on. And the space between you grows.

Sound familiar? You're not alone. Most couples struggle with communication after childbirth. Not because they don't love each other, but because no one ever taught them how to talk about sex, fear, exhaustion, or changing roles when a baby enters the picture. You both end up dancing around the issue— sometimes for months.

The good news? Honest, awkward, clumsy conversations are exactly what save intimacy. The bad news? Avoiding them is what turns small frustrations into full-blown resentments.

Let's talk about why silence hurts, how to break it without starting a fight, what scripts can help you start the hardest conversations, and why a partner's sensitivity makes all the difference.

Why silence is dangerous

You've probably heard the phrase "communication is key." It's true, but here's the kicker—silence is the lock. When you don't talk, assumptions take over.

- You think: "He must not find me attractive anymore."

- He thinks: "She doesn't want me. I must be doing something wrong."
- You both retreat.

One study showed that couples who communicate poorly about postpartum sex report lower relationship satisfaction and more sexual dysfunction months later. Silence doesn't protect you. It isolates you.

Checkpoint moment: If you've been avoiding the subject, it's not too late. Saying something—anything—is better than leaving the silence to do the talking.

The anatomy of a hard conversation

Okay, so how do you actually start? First, let's break it down. Good communication after baby has three steps:

1. **Timing**: Don't try to talk when you're half-asleep or during a crying fit. Pick a calm(ish) window—even if it's 15 minutes during a stroller walk.
2. **Tone**: Lead with honesty, not blame. "I'm scared it will hurt" lands better than "You never understand me."
3. **Truth**: Say the thing you've been avoiding, even if it comes out messy.

Sounds simple, right? But here's the thing: it's not natural. You've both been taught to protect each other from uncomfortable truths. This isn't about protecting. It's about connecting.

Case example: Danielle and Mark

Danielle, 33, avoided sex for three months after their son was born. Mark grew distant. Finally, she blurted out, "I'm terrified it's going to hurt, and I feel guilty every time you touch me." Mark admitted, "I thought you just weren't interested in me anymore."

Once they said the quiet parts out loud, things shifted. Mark stopped interpreting her hesitation as rejection. Danielle stopped hiding her fear. Together, they agreed to start with non-sexual intimacy—cuddling, back rubs—until she felt ready.

Lesson? Honesty often softens, not hardens, your partner's response.

Sample scripts to get started

Sometimes you need words when your brain goes blank. Here are some ready-to-use starters:

- "I want to be close to you, but I'm nervous about pain. Can we go slow together?"
- "I'm so tired that sex feels impossible right now. But I still want to connect. Can we try cuddling or massage?"
- "I feel different about my body. I need reassurance from you."
- "I miss you, but I don't know how to balance that with caring for the baby. Can we talk about it?"
- "I need to know that if I say stop, you'll stop. That will help me feel safer trying."

The magic isn't in perfect words—it's in the willingness to speak.

How partners can respond

Partners often feel helpless. They don't know if they should push, back off, or ignore the issue. Here's the deal: sensitivity and patience win every time.

- **Listen without fixing**: When your partner says, "I'm scared," don't jump to solutions. First say, "I hear you."
- **Reassure without pressure**: A gentle "I love you as you are" goes further than "We'll get through this" when it comes with expectation.
- **Be willing to adjust**: If sex feels out of reach, be open to other kinds of intimacy. Touch, affection, closeness—all count.
- **Check your own feelings**: Frustration is normal, but blaming or sulking creates distance. Express your feelings honestly: "I miss being close to you," not "You never want me."

Case example: **Ethan's mistake**
Ethan, 36, thought he was helping by saying, "Come on, it'll be fine. We just need to try." His wife, Maya, felt pressured and shut down even more. After counseling, Ethan learned to say instead, "What feels safe for you right now?" That simple change rebuilt trust.

Why emotional honesty builds desire

Here's a paradox: talking about sex openly doesn't kill desire—it grows it. Couples who can talk about fears and fantasies alike report higher satisfaction long-term. Why? Because intimacy isn't just bodies—it's safety. When you know you can say, "Stop," or, "I need slower," without being dismissed, your brain feels safe enough to engage sexually.

Safety equals openness. Openness equals desire.

Tools for real conversations

- **Use "I" statements**: Say, "I feel anxious," not "You make me anxious."
- **Pick a symbol**: Some couples choose a hand squeeze or word that means "pause." It turns scary moments into manageable ones.
- **Write it down**: If talking feels impossible, write a note. Sometimes written words feel safer.
- **Set a weekly check-in**: It doesn't have to be formal. Just ask: "How are you feeling about us?"

Case example: Priya and Amir

Priya, 30, said, "I don't know how to bring it up without crying." So she wrote Amir a letter: "I want you, but I'm scared. Please don't take my hesitation as rejection." Amir read it and felt relieved. They decided to have five-minute nightly check-ins after putting the baby down. Sometimes they talked about sex, sometimes just about how tired they were. But the regularity kept resentment from building.

Practical exercises for couples

1. **The compliment exchange**: Each day, tell each other one thing you appreciate. Doesn't have to be about appearance—gratitude builds intimacy.

2. **Touch without agenda**: Spend ten minutes touching—hands, shoulders, back—without moving to sex. The rule is: no expectation. This rewires safety.
3. **Two-minute truth**: Set a timer. Each partner talks uninterrupted for two minutes about how they feel. The other only listens. Switch. No fixing, just hearing.
4. **Code word for pause**: Agree on a word like "yellow." If sex feels overwhelming, say it. Partner stops. Trust grows.

Checkpoint reflection

Ask yourself: Have I been holding back from my partner because I'm scared of hurting their feelings—or mine? If yes, what's one sentence I could try tonight to open the door?

Key takeaways

- Silence breeds assumptions and distance. Honest words build safety.
- Timing, tone, and truth are the backbone of real conversations.
- Scripts can help when you don't know how to start.
- Partners who listen, reassure, and adjust create trust.
- Emotional safety fuels physical desire—openness is the real aphrodisiac.
- Simple exercises—like agenda-free touch or two-minute truth—keep communication alive.

Chapter 4: Knowing When Your Body Is Ready

Here's the truth most people won't tell you: just because your doctor says you're "cleared" doesn't mean your body (or your mind) is actually ready for sex. That little green light at the six-week check-up? It's a medical milestone, not an intimate one. And confusing the two is where so many couples hit trouble.

Healing after childbirth isn't about toughness, willpower, or ignoring discomfort. It's about paying attention to your body's signals, addressing pain or dryness before they turn into dread, and knowing when to ask for help. If you push too soon, intimacy can become linked with fear. If you wait too long without exploring gentle connection, you may feel stuck in avoidance.

This chapter is about finding that balance—understanding the real markers of readiness, what red flags to watch for, and how to gently rebuild comfort without pressure.

Why medical clearance isn't the whole story

At your postpartum check-up, your OB/GYN or midwife is mainly looking for:

- Is the uterus shrinking back to its pre-pregnancy size?
- Has vaginal bleeding stopped?
- Are stitches healing well?
- Is there any sign of infection?

If all those boxes are checked, you'll often hear, "You're cleared for normal activity, including sex." But let's stop there. What does "normal" even mean after childbirth? And whose definition are we using?

For some women, those physical milestones line up with how they feel. But for many, "clearance" comes long before the body feels safe, lubricated, or pain-free. Research shows that up to 50% of women report pain during sex three months after delivery, and 20% still report pain at six months.

So if you're cleared but not ready, you're not broken—you're human. Medical clearance is one piece. Comfort is the other.

Red flags that signal 'not yet'

Your body has ways of telling you it's not ready. Some are obvious, others are subtle. Pay attention to these signals:

- **Persistent pain**: Sharp, burning, or tearing sensations during attempts at sex.
- **Bleeding**: Any bleeding triggered by penetration or pressure.
- **Severe dryness**: Even with lubrication, sex feels abrasive.
- **Pelvic heaviness**: A dragging feeling in the vagina, which may indicate pelvic organ prolapse.
- **Fear or dread**: The body tensing up before touch, often an emotional sign tied to physical discomfort.

If any of these show up, that's not a sign to "push through." It's a sign to pause. Pain isn't a test of strength—it's information.

Why pain happens

Pain after childbirth can come from several sources:

- **Hormonal changes**: Low estrogen (especially while breastfeeding) thins vaginal tissues and reduces natural lubrication.
- **Scar tissue**: Tears, stitches, or C-section scars can create tightness or sensitivity.
- **Pelvic floor tension**: Muscles may over-contract in response to pain or fear, creating a cycle where they clamp down and make penetration more difficult.
- **Nerve sensitivity**: Nerves stretched during birth may take months to normalize.
- **Psychological anticipation**: If you expect pain, your body may tense, making pain more likely.

It's not "in your head." It's in your body. And your body and mind are in constant dialogue.

Case example: Rachel's roadblock

Rachel, 34, described sex at three months postpartum as "hitting a wall." Even with lubrication, penetration felt impossible. Her OB said everything looked fine. But Rachel's pelvic floor therapist discovered that scar tissue from a second-degree tear had healed too tightly. With scar mobilization and dilator therapy, Rachel gradually regained flexibility. By six months, she could have comfortable intercourse again.

The lesson? "Looking fine" on exam doesn't mean *feeling fine* during intimacy.

Comfort-first practices

So, what can you do while waiting for full readiness? Healing doesn't mean abstaining from intimacy altogether. It means redefining intimacy as comfort-first.

- **Use lubrication liberally**: Breastfeeding lowers estrogen, and dryness is normal. High-quality lubricants (water- or silicone-based) can reduce friction.
- **Try external touch first**: Hand-holding, cuddling, kissing, or massages rebuild closeness without pressure.
- **Explore non-penetrative pleasure**: Intimacy doesn't have to mean intercourse. Mutual touch, oral sex, or even lying together in skin contact count.
- **Check positions**: Side-lying or woman-on-top may reduce pressure compared to missionary. Pillows under the hips can also relieve strain.
- **Slow progression**: Start with short, playful encounters. Think of them as experiments, not performances.

Checkpoint: Notice the theme here? Comfort before performance. If you can approach intimacy with curiosity instead of pressure, you're already halfway there.

Pelvic floor therapy: a hidden key

Pelvic floor rehab isn't just about stopping leaks—it's about restoring pleasure. A therapist can assess muscle tone, scar mobility, and nerve sensitivity, then guide you through:

- **Breathing exercises** to relax overactive muscles.
- **Gentle stretches** to release tension.
- **Scar mobilization** to reduce tightness.
- **Gradual desensitization** using dilators.

Case example: **Hannah's surprise**
Hannah, 29, thought her pain was hormonal dryness. Lubricants

didn't help. Her pelvic therapist found that her muscles were locked in a guarding pattern. Once she learned to relax her pelvic floor with deep breathing and gentle stretches, her pain reduced dramatically.

The emotional side of readiness

Here's where it gets tricky. Sometimes your body is technically healed, but your emotions aren't. You may feel fear of pain, disconnection from your body, or resentment toward your partner. These are as real as physical barriers.

Ask yourself:

- Do I feel safe with my partner?
- Do I feel pressured?
- Do I feel resentful or unseen?
- Am I able to say "stop" without guilt?

If the answer is "no" to any of these, your readiness isn't just physical—it's relational. And it needs addressing.

Case example: Marisol's fear

Marisol, 27, had no physical complications. But each time her partner initiated sex, she froze. She realized she wasn't afraid of pain—she was afraid of disappointing him. Through counseling, she practiced saying, "Not now, but let's cuddle." That shift gave her the safety to try again later, on her terms. Desire followed once fear subsided.

Practical readiness checklist

Before trying penetrative sex, ask yourself:

1. Have I stopped bleeding completely?
2. Do I feel physically comfortable in daily activities (walking, lifting, sneezing)?
3. When I think about intimacy, do I feel curious rather than fearful?
4. Do I have strategies ready—lubrication, positions, communication—for comfort?
5. Am I willing to stop if it doesn't feel right?

If you answer "no" to any, you're still in the preparation stage. That's not failure—it's pacing.

Workbook-style exercise: comfort mapping

Draw three circles on a page. Label them:

- **Safe touch**: Types of touch you know feel good right now (hand-holding, massage).
- **Maybe touch**: Touch you're curious about but not sure (gentle breast play, kissing below the waist).
- **Not yet**: Touch that feels overwhelming (penetration, vigorous stimulation).

Update this map weekly. As your comfort grows, some "maybe" touches will shift to "safe."

When to seek professional help

Don't wait if you notice:

- Pain that persists beyond three months.
- Leakage that affects daily life.
- Fear so strong that you avoid all intimacy.
- Ongoing sadness, anxiety, or guilt around sex.

Pelvic floor therapists, OB/GYNs, sex therapists, and counselors all play a role. Healing isn't meant to be a solo project.

Checkpoint reflection

So here's the question: are you trying to force readiness because you think you "should"? Or are you listening to your body's actual signals? Because readiness isn't about pleasing a doctor, partner, or cultural timeline. It's about reclaiming safety and comfort.

Key takeaways

- Medical clearance doesn't equal readiness for sex. Comfort matters as much as healing.
- Pain, dryness, heaviness, or fear are red flags to pause, not push.
- Hormones, scar tissue, pelvic floor tension, and psychological anticipation all contribute to pain.
- Comfort-first intimacy—non-penetrative touch, lubrication, and slow progression—builds safety.
- Pelvic floor therapy can transform recovery by addressing hidden barriers.
- Emotional readiness matters as much as physical healing. Safety and trust are foundations.
- Readiness is personal. Your body sets the pace—not the calendar.

Chapter 5: Desire Rediscovered

Here's the blunt truth: after you've had a baby, desire doesn't just stroll back in like an old friend. For many women, it feels like it packed its bags, left a note on the fridge, and went into hiding. And if you're breastfeeding, sleep-deprived, or still healing, that missing spark can feel permanent. But it isn't. Desire isn't gone—it's just waiting for the right conditions to return.

This chapter isn't about forcing yourself to want sex. It's about rediscovering desire as something that grows when your body feels safe, your mind has room to breathe, and intimacy stops being a chore and becomes something you actually look forward to again.

Why desire disappears after baby

Let's stop blaming hormones alone. Yes, biology matters, but it's not the whole story. Desire is shaped by a mix of physical, emotional, and relational factors.

- **Hormones**: Prolactin (the milk-making hormone) rises while estrogen drops. That shift can reduce vaginal lubrication and lower libido.
- **Exhaustion**: Sleep deprivation suppresses dopamine and serotonin—both key to motivation and pleasure.
- **Body image**: If you don't like how you look or feel, it's hard to feel desirable.
- **Role overload**: You're a parent, partner, caregiver, maybe also working. Desire gets pushed to the bottom of the list.

- **Stress and resentment**: If you feel unsupported by your partner, desire turns into resistance.

Bottom line: if you don't feel rested, respected, or relaxed, desire won't show up. That's not brokenness. That's human wiring.

Case example: Anna's frustration

Anna, 30, said, "It's like my sex drive died. I don't miss it, but I miss *wanting it*." Her partner felt rejected. Anna blamed herself. In therapy, she realized that exhaustion and resentment were at the core. She felt like she carried 90% of the baby care, so sex felt like "one more demand." Once her partner started taking night shifts twice a week, Anna noticed something surprising— her desire crept back. It wasn't magic. It was energy plus balance.

Redefining what intimacy means

One of the traps after baby is equating intimacy with intercourse. If intercourse feels overwhelming, you may avoid all intimacy. That's a recipe for distance.

Let's expand the definition:

- Holding hands while walking
- Kissing without expectation
- Showering together
- Back rubs or massages
- Talking honestly without multitasking

When intimacy isn't reduced to "sex or nothing," desire has space to re-grow.

Checkpoint moment: Think about this—what small gestures make you feel connected? Write them down. You may realize desire starts in those everyday moments, not in the bedroom.

The science of responsive desire

Here's where most couples get it wrong. They assume desire should be spontaneous—you see your partner, you feel aroused, you act. That's true for some, but for many women, especially after childbirth, desire is **responsive**. It doesn't appear until you start engaging in touch or closeness.

In other words: you don't wait to feel turned on before trying. You try first, and desire builds as you go.

This doesn't mean forcing yourself into unwanted sex. It means giving yourself permission to explore small steps and see if arousal follows.

Case example: Lila's rediscovery

Lila, 33, thought she was "done with sex." Nothing about her husband sparked interest. But when they began a nightly ritual of massages with no agenda, she noticed that her body responded. She said, "I didn't want it at first. But once we started, desire woke up." This is responsive desire in action.

Exercises to rebuild desire

1. **Sensate focus**: Set aside 15 minutes for non-sexual touch. Focus on sensation, not performance. Caress arms, back, or face. The rule: no expectation of sex. This lowers pressure and awakens awareness.
2. **Fantasy exploration**: Desire often starts in the mind. Try journaling or talking with your partner about what scenarios or touches excite you.
3. **Mindfulness practice**: Spend 2–3 minutes focusing on your breath and body before intimacy. This calms the stress system and allows arousal to rise.
4. **Date-night plan**: Schedule time to be together outside the house, even if it's just coffee. Emotional closeness fuels physical desire.
5. **Pleasure mapping**: With your partner or alone, explore which parts of your body feel good now. Bodies change post-birth—pleasure spots may shift.

Practical supports

Sometimes simple aids make a big difference:

- **Lubricants and moisturizers**: Don't underestimate them. Breastfeeding dryness is real.
- **Position adjustments**: Woman-on-top or side-lying positions give you control and reduce discomfort.
- **Toys and aids**: Vibrators or dilators can help you reconnect with sensation at your own pace.
- **Scheduling**: It sounds unromantic, but planning intimacy ensures it doesn't get lost under diapers and dishes.

Case example: Monica and David

Monica, 29, and David hadn't had sex in four months. They felt more like co-parents than partners. Their therapist suggested scheduling "intimacy nights" with no expectation of intercourse. One night they played a board game and kissed on the couch. Another night they gave each other massages. Within weeks, desire returned—not because they forced it, but because they created space for it.

Emotional readiness and desire

Let's not forget: desire isn't only physical. It's deeply tied to how seen and supported you feel. Ask yourself:

- Do I feel emotionally connected to my partner?
- Do I feel supported in parenting duties?
- Do I feel safe expressing my needs without guilt?

If the answer is no, start there. Desire doesn't grow in resentment.

Workbook exercise: desire journal

Try keeping a short "desire journal." Each day, jot down:

- One moment I felt connected today was…
- One thing that made me feel cared for was…
- One type of touch I enjoyed (sexual or not) was…

Over time, you'll notice patterns. Maybe your desire sparks more after emotional closeness, or when you feel rested, or after laughter. These clues guide you toward conditions that nurture your libido.

Checkpoint reflection

Still with me? Here's the question: are you waiting for desire to show up on its own—or are you giving it a chance to grow by creating conditions for it?

Key takeaways

- Desire often fades after childbirth due to hormones, exhaustion, body image, and stress.
- Redefining intimacy beyond intercourse keeps connection alive.
- Responsive desire means arousal often follows touch, not precedes it.
- Exercises like sensate focus, pleasure mapping, and date nights rebuild desire step by step.
- Lubricants, position changes, and scheduling can ease the path.
- Emotional closeness and support are foundations for physical desire.
- Desire isn't gone—it's waiting for safety, energy, and connection to return.

Chapter 6: Pelvic Floor Rehab for Pleasure and Confidence

You've probably heard the phrase "Do your Kegels after birth." But that's about as useful as telling someone with a sprained ankle to "just walk it off." The pelvic floor is far more complex than a simple squeeze-and-release, and after childbirth it deserves more attention than most women are ever given.

This chapter is about more than stopping leaks or "tightening up." It's about restoring strength, flexibility, and awareness in a part of the body that directly impacts not only comfort but also confidence and pleasure. Done right, pelvic floor rehab helps you move through daily life without leaks, reduces pain during intimacy, and even heightens sexual satisfaction.

Why Pelvic Floor Rehab Matters

The pelvic floor is a group of muscles, ligaments, and connective tissue forming a supportive hammock at the base of your pelvis. These muscles hold up your bladder, uterus, and bowels. Childbirth—whether vaginal or cesarean—can stretch, strain, or injure this system.

Here's why rehab matters:

- **Improved sexual function**: Research shows that pelvic floor muscle training (PFMT) enhances desire, arousal, lubrication, orgasm, and reduces pain for postpartum women.
- **Better quality of life**: Multiple studies confirm that structured pelvic floor training improves both physical

and sexual health outcomes in the first year after childbirth.
- **Long-term protection**: PFMT lowers the risk of urinary incontinence and pelvic organ prolapse, common issues after pregnancy and delivery.

The goal isn't to get your body "back" to what it was, but to support what it needs now.

Case Study: Elena's Story

Elena, 29, passed her six-week check-up with no issues. But every time she laughed too hard, she leaked. Sex also felt tense and uncomfortable. Her OB told her it was "normal," but Elena didn't buy it.

A pelvic floor therapist assessed her and discovered her muscles weren't weak—they were overactive, constantly gripping in anticipation of pain. Through guided breathing, relaxation techniques, and gradual strengthening, Elena learned how to let go. Within weeks, her leaks improved, and intimacy no longer felt scary.

Her takeaway: the problem wasn't her body being "too loose," but her muscles being stuck.

Rehab Builds Pleasure and Confidence

Pelvic floor therapy isn't just about avoiding problems—it's about enhancing your intimate life.

- **Muscle balance**: Rehab teaches you both strength and relaxation. A muscle that can contract and release is a muscle that supports comfort and pleasure.
- **Increased circulation**: Exercises boost blood flow to the pelvic area, improving sensitivity and arousal.
- **Mind-body awareness**: Learning to notice subtle pelvic floor sensations helps you feel more connected to your body during intimacy.
- **Scar and nerve support**: Rehab techniques ease tightness and improve sensation in areas affected by tearing or surgery.

Case Study: Sarah's Breakthrough

Sarah, 32, avoided intimacy because of pressure and pain near her scar. She said, "I thought this was just how it would be forever." A pelvic therapist worked with her on scar tissue mobilization and gentle stretches. Within months, Sarah reported not only pain-free intimacy but stronger orgasms. "I finally didn't feel broken anymore," she said.

Exercises to Start With

You don't need equipment to begin. Here are four gentle practices to try:

1. **Breathing with Awareness**

- Lie on your back with knees bent.
- Inhale deeply, letting your belly expand.
- As you exhale, gently contract your pelvic floor (like you're stopping urine flow). Hold for 2–3 seconds.
- Release fully. Repeat 5–10 times.

2. **Pelvic Floor Release**

- Sit comfortably and breathe slowly.
- On each exhale, imagine your pelvic floor softening downward, like melting into the chair.
- Continue for 1–2 minutes.

3. **Scar Massage (when healed)**

- Place clean fingers on or near your scar.
- Gently move skin in circles or side-to-side.
- Notice if areas feel tight, numb, or sensitive.
- Continue for 2–3 minutes, stopping if painful.

4. **Confidence Control Exercise**

- If comfortable, insert a clean finger into the vagina.
- Try a gentle squeeze, then relax.
- Notice the difference between contraction and release.
- This builds awareness and confidence in how your muscles respond.

Workbook Exercise: Confidence Mapping

On a page, draw three circles:

- **Safe Zone**: Exercises or touches that feel comfortable (e.g., breathing, gentle massage).
- **Threshold Zone**: Sensations that bring slight tension but not pain (light internal awareness, scar touch).
- **Not Yet**: Anything that hurts or causes dread (penetration, high-pressure exercises).

Revisit this weekly. Over time, some "Not Yet" items will move into "Threshold," and eventually into "Safe."

Case Study: Maya's Healing

Maya, 27, hated her cesarean scar. She avoided touch near her belly and told her partner not to go near it during sex. Over time, her pelvic therapist encouraged her to use gentle self-massage to reconnect with sensation. Eventually, she allowed her partner to place a hand on her belly again. What began as discomfort became intimacy. For Maya, scar therapy wasn't just physical—it was emotional healing.

When to Seek Professional Help

Some things are best handled with guidance. Reach out to a pelvic floor therapist or your doctor if you notice:

- Pain during sex that doesn't improve with lubrication.
- Leaks during coughing, sneezing, or exercise.
- A heavy or dragging feeling in the vagina.
- Scar pain or sensitivity that makes intimacy difficult.
- Emotional distress tied to your pelvic health.

These aren't signs of weakness—they're signals. Getting help early prevents long-term frustration.

Checkpoint Reflection

Take a moment: how does your pelvic floor feel today? Do you sense tension, weakness, openness, or numbness? If you tried one of the exercises above, what did you notice? Write down one observation—even if it's, "I don't feel much yet." Awareness is the first step.

Key Takeaways

- Pelvic floor rehab is about restoring balance, not just strength.
- PFMT improves sexual function, reduces pain, and prevents long-term issues.
- Pain, leaks, or scar discomfort are not things to "tough out." They are treatable.
- Simple exercises—breathing, release, scar massage, gentle awareness—create powerful changes.
- Confidence comes from listening to your body and responding with care, not pressure.
- Professional support accelerates healing and restores intimacy.

Chapter 7: First Intimate Encounters

So here's the situation: you've made it through the storm of pregnancy, the marathon of labor, and the emotional rollercoaster of early postpartum recovery. Your body has been through stitches, swelling, hormones rising and crashing. You've adjusted to sleepless nights, endless feedings, and a new identity. Now, the world expects you to "get back" to intimacy. But the truth? That first time after childbirth is rarely smooth. It's awkward, unpredictable, sometimes funny, and sometimes frustrating. And that's okay.

This chapter is about learning how to approach first encounters with realism and compassion. You'll learn how to lower expectations, create a safe atmosphere, use positions that minimize discomfort, and rediscover intimacy through playfulness and patience—not pressure.

Setting expectations low

The biggest myth couples buy into is that sex will simply "resume" once you're medically cleared. Six weeks comes, you get a green light, and boom—back to normal. Not so fast.

Research shows that up to 83% of women experience pain during their first postpartum attempt at sex, and nearly half report ongoing discomfort for several months. Those numbers can feel discouraging, but they don't mean intimacy is doomed. They mean you need to reframe the goal.

Instead of "getting back to the way it was," think "discovering how it feels now." Instead of expecting fireworks, expect trial and error. Instead of demanding instant desire, expect gradual curiosity. This mindset reduces pressure on you and your partner and prevents disappointment from turning into resentment.

Checkpoint: Ask yourself—am I expecting perfection, or am I open to progress?

Creating a safe, comfortable atmosphere

Before you attempt intimacy, safety comes first. Why? Because arousal requires relaxation. If your brain is screaming "danger," your body won't respond.

Here's how to create a safe setting:

- **Communicate rules upfront**: Agree that you can stop anytime. Use a signal word if that feels easier. Safety increases trust, which increases openness.
- **Pick the timing**: Late at night when you're exhausted? Bad idea. Midday when the baby naps? Better. When you're somewhat rested, your body cooperates more.
- **Control the environment**: Dim lights, soft music, or simply a clean space. A chaotic environment adds to mental load.
- **Use supports**: Keep lubricant nearby. Vaginal dryness is common due to low estrogen during breastfeeding.

Case example: **Isabella and Tom**
Isabella dreaded her first time postpartum. She told Tom, "If it hurts, we stop." Tom agreed. They chose an afternoon when the baby was asleep, put on soft music, and focused on kissing. They didn't rush to penetration. Isabella later said, "The fact that I knew I could stop at any moment made me feel free enough to try."

Positions that reduce discomfort

Some positions are gentler than others during recovery. Start with ones that give you control and reduce deep pressure.

- **Side-lying (spooning)**: Both partners lie on their sides, facing the same way. Penetration is shallow, pressure is minimal, and you control movement.
- **Woman-on-top**: You set the depth, angle, and pace. Many women feel safer here because they can stop quickly if needed.
- **Modified missionary**: Place a pillow under your hips to reduce pelvic strain and allow comfort.
- **Rear-entry (gentle)**: Some find this position avoids pressure on sensitive areas, though it varies by comfort.

Case example: **Emily's adjustment**
Emily, 33, tried missionary first and burst into tears from the pain. She thought she had failed. Later, she tried woman-on-top and realized she could control the angle. It wasn't perfect, but it was manageable. That control gave her confidence to keep trying.

Using playfulness and patience

Here's the truth: your first time may feel clumsy. That doesn't mean failure—it means you're human. The best antidote to pressure is playfulness.

- **Laugh together**: If things feel awkward, embrace it. Humor defuses tension.
- **Focus on touch**: Don't make penetration the main event. Massage, kissing, oral sex—all count.

- **Breaks are allowed**: If something hurts, pause. Shift focus to cuddling or non-penetrative intimacy.
- **Celebrate small wins**: Even if sex isn't perfect, the fact that you tried is progress.

Case example: **Marta and Javier**
Marta said her first postpartum attempt was "a disaster." She leaked breast milk mid-encounter, which embarrassed her. Javier laughed and said, "Well, that's new!" Instead of ruining the moment, they both laughed, cleaned up, and cuddled. That levity kept intimacy alive rather than making it a traumatic memory.

Addressing common fears

- **Fear of pain**: Use plenty of lubrication, start with external touch, and go slow. Pain isn't weakness—it's feedback.
- **Fear of rejection**: Talk openly with your partner about your worries. Avoiding the subject creates more distance.
- **Fear of "not feeling sexy"**: Intimacy after childbirth isn't about appearance—it's about connection. Sexy is defined by closeness, not abs.

Practical steps for first encounters

1. Start with non-sexual intimacy (hugs, hand-holding).
2. Add sensual touch without pressure.
3. Use breathing techniques to relax pelvic muscles.
4. Experiment with positions that reduce pain.
5. Keep conversations open during the process.

Workbook Exercise: First Encounter Planner

Answer these before you try:

- What time of day do I feel most rested?
- Which positions feel safest to try first?
- What signal will I use if I want to stop?
- What non-sexual intimacy feels good right now?

Afterward, journal:

- How did I feel before we started?
- What worked better than I expected?
- What felt uncomfortable?
- One thing I'd like to try differently next time is…

Key takeaways

- The first postpartum encounter is about progress, not perfection.
- Safety, communication, and timing create the foundation for intimacy.
- Positions like side-lying and woman-on-top reduce pressure and increase control.
- Playfulness and patience turn awkward moments into connection.
- Fear is normal, but manageable when discussed openly.
- Planning ahead and reflecting afterward turns first attempts into learning experiences.

Chapter 8: When Things Don't Go Smoothly

Let's face it—sex after childbirth isn't always smooth sailing. You've read the books, maybe even practiced the exercises, and still, something feels off. Maybe intercourse is painful. Maybe your desire hasn't returned. Maybe your partner feels rejected, and the tension between you builds like a storm cloud. And if that's where you're at, you probably feel like you're failing. But here's the truth: you're not failing. You're normal.

This chapter is about what happens when intimacy doesn't fall back into place. We'll talk about painful sex, low libido, relationship tension, and what you can do about it. You'll hear real stories of couples who faced setbacks and found ways forward. You'll learn how to cope practically, when to seek help, and how to reframe these difficulties as part of the journey—not the end of it.

Painful sex

Pain during sex after childbirth—called dyspareunia—is extremely common. Studies show that up to 45% of women experience pain at three months postpartum, and about 20% still report pain a year later. Pain can feel sharp, burning, or like pressure. It can happen at penetration or linger afterward.

Causes include:

- **Vaginal dryness** due to low estrogen, especially while breastfeeding.
- **Scar tissue** from tears, stitches, or cesarean incisions.

- **Pelvic floor muscle tension**—muscles clench as a protective response to pain.
- **Psychological anticipation**—fear of pain leads to tension, which creates more pain.

What helps:

- **Lubricants**: Choose a high-quality water- or silicone-based lube. Reapply often.
- **Moisturizers**: Vaginal moisturizers can help keep tissues supple.
- **Pelvic floor therapy**: A therapist can release scar tissue, teach relaxation, and restore muscle balance.
- **Hormone support**: Low-dose estrogen creams (prescribed) can improve dryness in breastfeeding women.
- **Communication**: Tell your partner honestly what hurts and when to stop.

Case example: **Holly's frustration**
Holly, 28, tried to have sex at 12 weeks postpartum. She cried from the burning pain. Her partner felt helpless, and she avoided intimacy for months. Finally, she saw a pelvic floor therapist who found scar tissue pulling at her perineum. With massage and exercises, Holly regained comfort. "I thought I'd never enjoy sex again. I was wrong—it just took help."

Low libido

If your sex drive feels nonexistent, you're not alone. Studies suggest that 50–80% of new mothers experience low desire in the first year postpartum.

Why does libido tank?

- **Exhaustion**: Sleep deprivation wipes out dopamine, the brain's reward chemical.
- **Hormones**: Prolactin (milk production) suppresses estrogen, reducing arousal.
- **Body image**: If you dislike how your body looks, desire plummets.
- **Role overload**: Caring for a baby, managing a household, and working leaves little mental energy.
- **Resentment**: If you feel unsupported, desire gets replaced by irritation.

Here's the kicker: for many women, desire isn't spontaneous—it's **responsive**. That means it appears once intimacy begins, not before. If you wait to "feel in the mood" before starting, you may wait forever. If you start small—touch, massage—desire may follow.

Case example: **Naomi's rediscovery**
Naomi, 34, said, "I didn't crave sex, but once we started cuddling, my body remembered what it liked." She shifted her mindset from "I should feel desire first" to "Let's see what happens." That change opened the door to arousal.

Tension in the relationship

Intimacy issues ripple into the relationship. Partners may misinterpret avoidance as rejection. You may feel pressured, creating a cycle of distance.

- **The partner's view**: They may think, "She doesn't want me anymore," or "I'm not attractive to her."
- **Your view**: You may think, "He doesn't get it," or "I can't handle one more demand."
- **The outcome**: Silence builds resentment. Resentment builds distance.

Checkpoint: Have you both said out loud what's really going on? Or are you guessing what the other feels?

Case example: **Rachel and Omar**
Rachel avoided sex after painful attempts. Omar grew angry, interpreting it as rejection. In therapy, Rachel admitted her fear of tearing again. Omar admitted his fear of losing their bond. By naming fears, they rebuilt trust. Slowly, with guidance, sex stopped being a battlefield and became something they approached together.

Practical coping steps

1. **Reframe setbacks**: Instead of "We failed," say "We learned what doesn't work today."
2. **Expand intimacy**: Don't limit closeness to intercourse. Holding hands, kissing, cuddling—all count.
3. **Schedule connection**: A planned time for affection reduces the "we never connect" problem.
4. **Use humor**: Laughing at awkward moments keeps intimacy light.
5. **Focus on safety**: Agree that either partner can pause or stop anytime without guilt.

When to seek help

Don't wait if:

- Pain continues beyond three months despite basic adjustments.
- You feel no desire *and* no enjoyment once intimacy starts.
- Relationship tension feels constant.

- Anxiety or depression affect your connection.

Who to see:

- **Pelvic floor therapists** for pain, leaks, or scar issues.
- **OB/GYNs** for hormonal or medical concerns.
- **Sex therapists** for desire, communication, or emotional barriers.
- **Couples' counselors** for ongoing conflict.

Case example: **Leah and Ben**
Leah avoided sex for nearly a year. Ben felt shut out. They entered therapy, where Leah admitted untreated postpartum depression was crushing her desire. With treatment, her mood improved, and intimacy gradually returned. "We didn't just fix our sex life," Ben said. "We fixed how we talk about everything."

Real stories of setbacks and breakthroughs

- **Megan's tears**: "I thought we were ready. It hurt so much, I cried in the bathroom. My husband felt awful. But we tried again weeks later with lube and different positions, and it was better. Not perfect, but better."
- **Julia's numbness**: Julia, 26, had a cesarean. Her scar felt numb, and she hated being touched. With scar massage guided by a therapist, sensation slowly returned. She said, "Touching there used to feel alien. Now it feels like me again."
- **Sasha's resentment**: Sasha felt like her partner didn't help enough with the baby. Sex became the last thing she wanted. After renegotiating household duties, she said, "Desire came back once I wasn't carrying everything alone."

Workbook Exercise: Coping Reflection

1. Which intimacy challenge feels hardest for me right now—pain, low libido, or tension?
2. What have I tried so far, and what worked even a little?
3. What signals from my body or emotions tell me I'm not ready?
4. What support—partner, therapist, medical—do I need next?
5. One step I can take this week to reduce pressure is...

Checkpoint reflection

Ask yourself: am I treating setbacks as permanent failures, or as part of the process? Because intimacy after childbirth isn't linear. It's trial and error, progress and pauses.

Key takeaways

- Pain, low libido, and relationship tension are common but treatable.
- Pain signals deserve attention—don't push through.
- Desire is often responsive, not spontaneous.
- Silence breeds resentment—honesty builds trust.
- Humor, safety, and small steps ease pressure.
- Professional support accelerates healing and restores connection.

Chapter 9: Keeping Intimacy Alive in Parenthood

So here's the deal: parenthood is exhausting. You've got diapers, late-night feedings, work deadlines, school schedules, and about a hundred "urgent" things that eat into your day. By the time the house is quiet, you're not exactly in the mood for romance—you're in the mood for sleep. Sound familiar? Of course it does. For many couples, intimacy becomes the first thing to vanish once a baby arrives.

But here's the truth—you *can* keep intimacy alive while raising kids. It won't look like it did before. It won't always feel glamorous. And no, it doesn't mean a wild sex life every night (unless you're one of the rare unicorns who pulls that off). What it does mean is creating a conscious effort to nurture closeness, passion, and fun so that your bond as partners doesn't get lost under the weight of parenthood.

This chapter tackles how to sustain intimacy when everything else seems more urgent. We'll talk about scheduling sex without killing spontaneity, creative alternatives when you're too tired, and long-term rituals that keep love alive.

Why intimacy is often the first thing to vanish

Let's start with the obvious: intimacy slips away because you're both tired, overwhelmed, and operating in survival mode. Sleep deprivation alone has been linked to lower sexual satisfaction and decreased relationship quality. Add in hormonal changes, body image concerns, and the sheer logistics of parenting, and intimacy often falls to the bottom of the list.

But here's something people rarely admit—sometimes couples let intimacy slide because they *assume* it will naturally bounce back later. The problem? Later never comes. Habits form quickly. If you let avoidance become the pattern, you risk drifting apart emotionally and physically.

Case example: **Diana and Luis**
Diana, 32, told me, "We thought this was just a phase. But after two years, sex was still rare, and we felt like roommates." They finally realized that intimacy doesn't just return on its own—it has to be chosen, nurtured, and sometimes scheduled.

Scheduling sex without killing spontaneity

You might cringe at the idea of "scheduled sex." It sounds clinical, like booking a dentist appointment. But here's the reality—without planning, it often doesn't happen at all. Couples who make intimacy intentional report greater satisfaction because they carve out protected space for each other.

How to make scheduling feel sexy, not sterile:

- **Think of it as anticipation, not obligation**: Knowing a date night is coming can build excitement.
- **Keep it flexible**: If you're both exhausted, reschedule without guilt.
- **Make it ritual-based**: Maybe Saturday mornings become cuddle-and-coffee-in-bed time. Maybe Thursday nights mean no phones after 9 p.m.
- **Frame it positively**: Instead of "We *have* to do this," try "We *get* to focus on us."

Quick tip: Put it on your shared calendar. Treat it like an important appointment. Because honestly, it is.

Creative alternatives when you're too tired for intercourse

Sometimes, you'll be too drained for a full-on sexual encounter. That doesn't mean intimacy is off the table. Intimacy is broader than intercourse—it's any activity that makes you feel close, connected, and desired.

Ideas for low-energy connection:

- **Extended cuddling**: Skin-to-skin releases oxytocin, the bonding hormone
- **Massage exchange**: Trade five-minute massages before bed.
- **Sensual, not sexual touch**: Run fingers through each other's hair, hold hands, spoon.
- **Make-out sessions**: Remember when kissing alone felt electric? Bring that back.
- **Shared bath or shower**: Even if it doesn't lead to sex, it restores physical closeness.
- **Erotic reading or watching together**: Sometimes desire builds by sharing erotic material in a safe, playful way.

Case example: **Harper and Jae**
Harper confessed, "I dreaded sex because I was too tired. But when Jae suggested just cuddling and giving each other massages, the pressure disappeared. And funny enough, sometimes that led to more. Sometimes it didn't. Both felt okay."

Long-term connection rituals

Quick check-in: How often do you and your partner connect outside of parenting roles? If the answer is "rarely," you need rituals. Rituals anchor your relationship, even when life feels chaotic.

Ideas for connection rituals:

- **Daily check-in**: Five minutes each night to ask, "What was the hardest part of your day? What was the best part?"
- **Weekly date night**: Even if it's just Netflix and takeout at home, commit to it.
- **Monthly adventure**: Try a new restaurant, hike, or class together once a month.
- **Inside jokes**: Humor strengthens bonds. Keep your private language alive.
- **Touch habit**: A hug every morning and kiss every night—non-negotiable.

Case example: **Maya and Tom**
They started a ritual of "Sunday morning pancakes in bed" after their first child was born. It became sacred. They'd eat, laugh, and sometimes fool around. Years later, their kids joke about it, but Maya and Tom swear it's one reason their intimacy stayed alive.

Barriers to keeping intimacy alive

Let's be real. There are roadblocks.

- **Resentment**: If one partner feels they carry more of the parenting load, desire disappears.
- **Technology**: Phones in bed kill more intimacy than people admit.
- **Comparison**: Social media creates unrealistic expectations about "perfect couples."

- **Shame**: Feeling unattractive can make you avoid closeness altogether.

Checkpoint: Which barrier affects you most right now? Naming it is step one to fixing it.

Strategies to rebuild intimacy in parenthood

1. **Divide responsibilities fairly**: Nothing kills desire faster than resentment over chores.
2. **Create child-free moments**: Even 15 minutes after bedtime counts.
3. **Limit technology**: Phones out of the bedroom. Seriously.
4. **Work on body confidence**: Exercise, self-care, or therapy can help restore comfort in your skin.
5. **Celebrate small wins**: Did you cuddle instead of collapsing into bed? That counts.

Case stories of long-term success

- **Anna and Jacob**: After their second baby, sex dwindled. Anna felt resentful, Jacob felt unwanted. They implemented "date night Thursdays" and divided chores equally. Within months, their closeness returned. Anna said, "I don't feel like his mother anymore. I feel like his partner again."
- **Claire and Devin**: Claire hated her postpartum body. Devin reassured her, but she avoided intimacy anyway. Therapy helped Claire confront body shame, and intimacy slowly returned. She said, "I realized my partner never stopped desiring me. I just stopped desiring myself."

- **Sofia and Malik**: They created a ritual of morning coffee together before the kids woke up. No phones, just talking. Sofia said, "It's five minutes, but it sets the tone for the whole day."

Workbook Exercise: Intimacy Audit

Take 10 minutes together to answer:

1. How often do we connect physically each week (sex, cuddling, kissing)?
2. How often do we connect emotionally (talking, laughing, checking in)?
3. What barriers are getting in our way most often?
4. Which one small ritual could we start this week to feel closer?
5. What's one thing I need from my partner that I haven't voiced?

Reflection prompt

Ask yourself: Are we letting intimacy vanish because we think parenthood makes it impossible, or because we haven't chosen to prioritize it?

Key takeaways

- Intimacy often disappears in parenthood due to fatigue, stress, and assumptions.
- Scheduling sex isn't unromantic—it's strategic.

- Closeness doesn't always mean intercourse; alternatives matter.
- Connection rituals protect your relationship from drifting into roommate territory.
- Honest division of responsibilities and body confidence play huge roles in desire.
- Small, consistent efforts create long-term intimacy.

Chapter 10: Tools, Resources, and Exercises

By now, you've heard the stories, absorbed the research, and wrestled with some uncomfortable truths about postpartum intimacy. You've seen how physical healing, emotional shifts, and relationship changes can all pile on to make sex after baby a complicated, sometimes frustrating process. But here's the part that makes the difference between "knowing" and actually "doing": tools and practice.

This last section is about putting everything together into something you and your partner can *use*—not just read about and forget. You'll find journal prompts, practical exercises, couple rituals, and a curated set of resources to keep you supported after you close this book. Think of this chapter as your toolkit. When things get tough (and they will), you'll have a set of practices to lean on.

Why structured tools matter

Here's the thing. Willpower and "good intentions" don't sustain intimacy. You need systems. Rituals. Tangible practices. Research shows that couples who intentionally build intimacy routines—like touch rituals, communication check-ins, or planned intimacy—report stronger bonds and higher satisfaction.

And here's another truth: postpartum challenges don't resolve overnight. Tools like journaling, structured intimacy dates, and touch exercises aren't "extras"—they're maintenance for your relationship. Just like your body needs physical rehab after childbirth, your connection needs structured attention too.

Journal prompts to track progress

Writing is one of the simplest but most powerful tools for self-awareness. When you write, you notice patterns, acknowledge emotions, and clarify what you really need. These prompts are designed for new mothers but can be adapted for partners too.

Prompts to start with:

- *How do I currently feel about my body? What words come up most often when I describe it to myself?*
- *What intimacy do I miss most right now? Is it sex, cuddling, flirting, or something else?*
- *What fears do I hold about resuming sex?*
- *What small sign of progress have I noticed this week?*
- *What do I want my partner to know but haven't said yet?*
- *How do I want intimacy to look three months from now?*

Set aside 10–15 minutes once or twice a week to answer one. Don't overthink it—just write what comes out. Over time, these entries become a map of your healing.

Case example: **Elena**
Elena, a new mom, started journaling about her fear that her C-section scar made her "unattractive." Weeks later, she noticed her language shifting: "My body is softer, yes, but it's also stronger." The act of writing showed her gradual mindset change, something she hadn't noticed day-to-day.

Couple's intimacy dates

Date nights often get sidelined in early parenthood. But you don't need fancy dinners or babysitters every week to reconnect.

You need structured *intimacy dates*—time focused on building closeness, not just logistics or Netflix.

Ideas for intimacy dates:

1. **Sensory night**: Light candles, use massage oil, explore each other's senses with touch, taste, and smell.
2. **Memory lane**: Revisit early photos, tell each other what first attracted you.
3. **Gratitude exchange**: Write three things you love about each other and read them out loud.
4. **Desire check-in**: Ask, "What kind of intimacy do you want more of right now—sexual, emotional, playful?"
5. **Adventure at home**: Try cooking a new dish together, dancing in the kitchen, or playing a game that sparks laughter.

Why these work: anticipation builds, novelty stimulates desire, and you carve out intentional space for each other.

Case example: **Maya and Sam**
Maya and Sam started a "Friday night intimacy ritual." Sometimes it was sex, sometimes just back rubs and talking. Maya said, "It became our anchor. No matter how chaotic the week was, we knew we had that night for us."

Massage and touch exercises

Touch is one of the fastest ways to rekindle closeness. It doesn't always have to be sexual. In fact, removing the expectation of sex often makes touch feel safer and more inviting.

Try this exercise:

- **Set the scene**: Quiet room, warm lighting, no phones.

- **Trade roles**: One person receives for five minutes, then switch.
- **Focus on nonsexual zones**: Shoulders, back, arms, scalp, feet.
- **Use slow, intentional movements**. Pay attention to how your partner reacts.
- **Communicate**: Use simple phrases like "more pressure," "slower," or "that feels good."

Advanced variation: Try sensate focus—a therapeutic exercise where you explore each other's bodies without aiming for orgasm. The goal is rediscovering sensation and connection. This approach has been shown to help couples struggling with postpartum desire and performance anxiety.

Resource list

Sometimes you need outside guidance. Here's a curated set of resources to support ongoing intimacy after childbirth.

- **Pelvic floor therapy**: Find a licensed pelvic floor physiotherapist through professional organizations (e.g., American Physical Therapy Association, Pelvic Health section).
- **Sex therapy directories**: The American Association of Sexuality Educators, Counselors, and Therapists (AASECT) offers certified provider listings.
- **Postpartum support groups**: Postpartum Support International (PSI) hosts free groups and connects parents with local counselors.
- **Books worth exploring**:
    - *Come As You Are* by Emily Nagoski – on women's sexual desire and context.
    - *The Fourth Trimester* by Kimberly Ann Johnson – holistic postpartum healing.

     o *Reclaiming Desire* by Barry & Emily McCarthy – couples navigating mismatched libido.
- **Apps and tools**: Guided meditation apps (like Headspace or Insight Timer) have intimacy and relationship tracks that couples can use.

Workbook activity: Intimacy goals planner

Sit down together and write out:

1. One emotional goal (e.g., "Talk about our feelings once a week").
2. One physical goal (e.g., "Cuddle three nights a week").
3. One sexual goal (e.g., "Try sex at least once this month, no pressure").
4. One fun goal (e.g., "Dance in the living room once this week").

Put these somewhere visible (fridge, bathroom mirror) as a gentle reminder.

Reflection prompt

Ask yourself: Which of these tools feels most natural for me to start today? Which feels like it will stretch me in a good way?

Key takeaways

- Tools matter because intimacy doesn't happen by accident—it's cultivated.

- Journaling helps you notice emotional shifts and track healing.
- Intimacy dates bring back anticipation and novelty.
- Touch exercises restore comfort and connection without pressure.
- Resources like therapy, books, and support groups provide backup when you need it.
- Setting small, realistic goals keeps you moving forward without overwhelm.

Appendix: Tools for Postpartum Intimacy

Postpartum Body Journal
(Use this to track physical healing, sensations, and readiness.)

- Date: _____
- Physical symptoms I noticed today (pain, dryness, fatigue, pelvic heaviness):
  _____
- Things that helped (rest, hydration, stretching, pelvic floor exercise, medication, other):
  _____
- Body comfort rating (0 = very uncomfortable, 10 = completely comfortable): _____
- Notes for next week's check-in:
  _____

Emotional Check-In Log
(Weekly reflection on mood, self-image, and intimacy readiness.)

- Week of: _____
- Emotions I experienced most often this week:
  _____
- Did I feel connected to my partner? (Yes / No / Sometimes)
- How did "mom guilt" or stress affect me?
  _____
- What made me feel good about myself this week?
  _____

- One intention for next week:
  _____

Couple's Communication Starter Cards
(Print, cut, and use in short conversations with your partner.)

- One thing I need from you this week is…
- One way I'd like to connect outside of sex is…
- My biggest worry about intimacy right now is…
- One compliment I want to hear from you is…
- Something I miss from before the baby that we can bring back is…

Pelvic Floor Tracker
(Daily record of strengthening and awareness exercises.)

- Date: _____
- Kegel holds: _____ seconds × _____ reps
- Breathing with relaxation: Done / Not Done
- Stretch or yoga for pelvic release: Yes / No
- Any discomfort during exercise:
  _____
- Confidence rating (0 = no confidence, 10 = strong confidence): _____

Intimacy Date Planner
(A structured but fun way to keep closeness alive.)

- This week's date idea: _____
- Time and place: _____

- Will intimacy involve: Touch / Conversation / Play / Sex / Other
- Boundaries or limits we agree on:

  _____

- One thing I hope to feel by the end:

  _____

First Intimate Encounter Checklist

(For easing into physical intimacy after clearance from your provider.)

- Am I pain-free enough to try? □ Yes □ No
- Do I have lubrication nearby? □ Yes □ No
- Have we set aside quiet time (no interruptions)? □ Yes □ No
- Do I feel safe saying "pause" or "stop"? □ Yes □ No
- Comfortable positions planned? □ Yes □ No
- Gentle agreement with partner: "Progress, not perfection." □ Yes □ No

---

Setback Recovery Log

(For days when sex is painful, or libido feels gone.)

- Date: _____
- What happened: _____
- My feelings: _____
- How my partner responded:

  _____

- Coping strategy I tried (rest, communication, therapy tools, etc.): _____
- Did it help? □ Yes □ No □ A little
- One thing to try differently next time:

  _____

Connection Rituals Checklist
(Daily and weekly habits to strengthen closeness.)

- Daily 5-minute cuddle (without phones): □ Done
- Shared laugh or inside joke today: □ Done
- Check-in question: "How are you, really?" □ Done
- Weekly couple's meeting (schedule, stress, needs): □ Done
- Shared relaxation (bath, walk, music): □ Done

Resource Notes Page
(Record contact details for quick access.)

- OB/GYN or midwife: _____
- Pelvic floor therapist: _____
- Couples' counsellor or sex therapist:
  _____
- Local postpartum support group:
  _____
- Online community or resource:
  _____

Closing Reflection

- What has changed for me since starting this book?
  _____
- How do I now define intimacy (beyond sex)?
  _____
- What are the three biggest lessons I want to carry forward?
  1. _____

2. _____

3. _____

_____

Reference

- Barrett, G., Pendry, E., Peacock, J., Victor, C., Thakar, R., & Manyonda, I. (2000). Women's sexual health after childbirth. *BJOG: An International Journal of Obstetrics & Gynaecology*, 107(2), 186–195.
- Brotto, L. A., Basson, R., & Luria, M. (2008). A mindfulness-based group psychoeducational intervention targeting sexual arousal disorder in women. *Journal of Sexual Medicine*, 5(7), 1646–1659.
- De Judicibus, M. A., & McCabe, M. P. (2002). Psychological factors and the sexuality of pregnant and postpartum women. *Journal of Sex Research*, 39(2), 94–103.
- Dekel, S., Stuebe, C., & Dishy, G. (2017). Childbirth-induced posttraumatic stress syndrome: A systematic review of prevalence and risk factors. *Frontiers in Psychology*, 8, 560.
- Field, T. (2010). Postpartum depression effects on early interactions, parenting, and safety practices: A review. *Infant Behavior and Development*, 33(1), 1–6.
- Glazener, C. M. (1997). Sexual function after childbirth: Women's experiences, persistent morbidity, and lack of professional recognition. *BJOG: An International Journal of Obstetrics & Gynaecology*, 104(3), 330–335.
- Harlow, B. L., Wise, L. A., & Stewart, E. G. (2001). Prevalence and predictors of chronic lower genital tract discomfort. *American Journal of Obstetrics and Gynecology*, 185(3), 545–550.
- Hirsch, M., & Bhattacharya, S. (2015). Sexual function after childbirth. *Best Practice & Research Clinical Obstetrics & Gynaecology*, 29(1), 116–127.
- Hodnett, E. D., Gates, S., Hofmeyr, G. J., & Sakala, C. (2013). Continuous support for women during childbirth. *Cochrane Database of Systematic Reviews*, (7), CD003766.

- Leeman, L., & Rogers, R. (2012). Sex after childbirth: Postpartum sexual function. *Obstetrics and Gynecology Clinics of North America*, 39(3), 559–571.
- Leeman, L., Rogers, R. G., Borders, N., Teaf, D., Qualls, C., & Fullilove, A. M. (2016). Effect of perineal laceration and repair technique on postpartum sexual function. *Journal of Midwifery & Women's Health*, 61(4), 427–434.
- McDonald, E. A., & Brown, S. J. (2013). Does method of birth make a difference to when women resume sex after childbirth? *BJOG: An International Journal of Obstetrics & Gynaecology*, 120(7), 823–830.
- McDonald, S. D., Pullenayegum, E., Chapman, B., Sword, W., Foster, G., Vera, C., & Karovitch, A. (2015). Prevalence and predictors of sexual problems after childbirth. *Obstetrics & Gynecology*, 125(3), 683–691.
- Rosen, R., Brown, C., Heiman, J., Leiblum, S., Meston, C., Shabsigh, R., ... & Ferguson, D. (2000). The Female Sexual Function Index (FSFI): A multidimensional self-report instrument for the assessment of female sexual function. *Journal of Sex & Marital Therapy*, 26(2), 191–208.
- World Health Organization. (2013). *WHO Recommendations on Postnatal Care of the Mother and Newborn*. Geneva: WHO.

www.ingramcontent.com/pod-product-compliance
Lightning Source LLC
Chambersburg PA
CBHW070916280326
41934CB00008B/1752